If I eat carbs and sugar my energy level and mood
will drop dramatically and my sense of anxiety will
increase.

When I eat non-keto foods, they attack me physically.

I love being keto-adapted and will eat this way for life.

Eating something less bad than something else is not helpful.

Only by being aware of the truth of Keto can I enjoy the freedom to living that brings.

I understand that glucose is impacted by sleep, exercise, inflammation and stress, and I will keep that in consideration when trying to understand my glucose levels.

I will put the oxygen mask on me first by eating in a way that makes me feel good.

I have control over my feelings, thoughts, and choices daily.

Everything I eat nourishes and strengthens my body and mind.

If I eat carbs and sugar I will want to eat more and more carbs and sugar.

I am not afraid to say no when I need to.

My body was never designed to handle wheat, grains, starches, carbs, and sugar.

I have a strong body

I eat well and exercise to enjoy lasting good health

I will become healthy in mind and body

I don't aim for perfection. I accept mistakes and learn from them.

I am attracting health into my life

Eating high fat, moderate protein and low carb is the best thing I can do for my well-being.

Fat is the only thing that will satiate my hunger and turn off the cravings.

I will recognize addict thinking…rationalizations no different than mental patients who feel good when they take medicine and then decide they don't need medicine.

I vow to never give up and be true to what works.

I accept the past and know the future will be bright and happy.

I will recognize that when I do feel good that is not an acceptable excuse to have wheat, grains, starches, carbs and sugar.

I look forward to achieving my ideal weight. I will wear.....and enjoy.......

I am naturally healthy

Without judgment, I will simply return to the path if I fall off.

My mind is healthy

Glucose spikes cause cravings that can never be satisfied.

If I should get hungry, there are no exceptions
–physically or socially—where eating wheat, grains,
carbs will be helpful.

My path is to remain curious, search for the truth through N=1 tests and accept the reality that truth reveals.

Only my glucose level can tell me if my food and diet choices are working to keep me healthy (not my rationalizations), so I will test as needed.

My medicine is healthy, whole foods and a new understanding of what works.

It's not that I can't eat anything that I want. I'm making the healthy choice not to.

I accept that I have a problem with wheat, grains, starches, carbs and sugar.

I will not judge myself if I fall off the path.

By keeping low glucose levels I cannot go into keto-acidosis and any fear of ketoacidosis is residual defense mechanism.

I am a fat burning machine.

It does not matter what other people say or do. What matters is how I choose to react and what I choose to believe about myself.

I enjoy eating a ketogenic diet and have no desire to cheat as I know it make me feel better than any other way of eating.

I do not need carbs.